Healing Leaky Gut
TAKE YOUR LIFE BACK THROUGH NUTRITION AND HEALTHY LIVING

Sage M. Howard

Copyright © 2016 Sage M. Howard

nutritionandhealthyliving.org

All rights reserved.

ISBN: 1533662142
ISBN-13: 978-1533662149

DISCLAIMER

This guide is intended for educational purposes only and should not be taken as medical advice. Please consult with your primary health provider before attempting the guidelines in this book. We cannot be held responsible for any application of this information.

Any third-party companies, websites and people mentioned in this book are not directly affiliated in any way with us and we cannot be held responsible for any actions, methods or ideas that they may promote, or vice-versa.

CONTENTS

	Introduction	I
1	What is Leaky Gut	1
2	Diagnosing Leaky Gut	7
3	How to Heal Naturally	9
4	Important Concepts	20
5	Sleep, Exercise and Reducing Stress	23
6	Supplements	26
7	Candida	29
8	Depression and Anxiety	32
9	Living After Leaky Gut	34
10	Believing in Yourself	36
	Conclusion	37
	Extras	38
	About the Author	41

INTRODUCTION

Four years ago I began my healing journey. It wasn't without provoking, though. I was a freshman in college, struggling to even get to class, let alone trying to get good grades. I had decided I would give a new doctor one last chance. Someone I had heard so many great things about. I scheduled the appointment and awaited the day I would finally know what was wrong with me, and how to finally get better.

After taking a basic blood sample, the doctor asked me what was wrong. After explaining the debilitating abdominal pain, fevers, uncomely bowel movements, passing out, exhaustion, brain fog, slow heart-beat, multiple allergies, asthma, anemia, and the rest of the problems on my list, he told me it sounded like I had depression and all of my problems were caused by it. He offered to give me depression meds. I sat there dumbfounded for a moment then I leveled with him telling him I was a psychology major and I knew without a doubt that my problems were not caused by depression. They were more likely the cause. He relaxed a little, told me to keep an eye on "it" and to come back in four months if I hadn't gotten better by then.

I left frustrated feeling like my problems had landed on deaf ears, frustrated that the doctor everybody raved about didn't have a clue. I knew from that moment forward the only person who could change my situation was me. I couldn't wait another four months. I was desperate. I knew that the only one who cared as much about my health was me, and I knew I had to take healing into my own hands. So at that moment I decided to change my health, to change my life. And I did.

The irony? Four months later I *was* healed, permanently. And you can heal too.

1 WHAT IS LEAKY GUT

Leaky Gut is reported to be found (in some degree or another) in roughly 80% of all adults in America. That's no small number. Leaky Gut Syndrome goes by many names, including Irritable Bowel Syndrome, Celiac Disease, Intolerances of any kind and adult food allergies. I'm not saying that all of these instances are cases of Leaky Gut, but they usually are.

"Leaky Gut Syndrome" is the name for what happens when your digestive system becomes inflamed and the intestines in your body become "semi-permeable," meaning that certain objects are allowed to pass through into your blood stream, including food particles and toxins.

Understand that *the intestines should never, ever allow objects to pass through them*. When food passes through into your blood stream, it is attacked.

Your body creates anti-bodies against these toxins, even if they are normal food particles, because they are foreign to your bloodstream. Any item in your bloodstream that doesn't belong is called an "antigen." Your body attacks these antigens and purges them from your system. It will purge them through diarrhea, throwing up, acne, hives, and many other ways, usually resulting in a violent sickness.

This is also the exact cause of a food sensitivity or "food allergy." Food allergies are not normal in adults and are almost always caused by Leaky Gut. Celiac disease is another instance of this food sensitivity.

Causes

Leaky Gut is caused by inflammation in the digestive system. This is usually caused by:

Antibiotics – These kill off all good and bad bacteria in your digestive system. Without probiotics to restore the good bacteria, the bad bacteria is allowed to multiply and overwhelm the digestive system. This causes the intestines to become inflamed and creates a semi-permeable layer in your intestines.

Poor Diet – Processed foods have a lot of preservatives, chemicals and toxins that create inflammation and semi-permeability in the intestines. Fast food isn't the worst thing in the world, but food like that every day can kill you. I'd suggest watching "Super-Size Me." That might dissuade you from eating fast food.

Birth control – This is actually a very common cause of Leaky Gut in women. Birth control changes the chemistry of a woman's body and can cause hormonal imbalance. This creates an imperfect environment for the body and can cause a lot of stress in the digestive system. Stress causes inflammation and that causes Leaky Gut. Birth control can contain many dangerous toxins which also add to creating leaky gut.

Medication – Contrary to popular belief, most medication is actually doing you more harm than it is good. While some people may need to take certain medications to stay alive, dependencies should be avoided and overcome if possible. Medication can contain many harmful substances that also create inflammation in the intestines which causes the semi-permeability. Many medications also disturb the body's natural order which can cause malfunctions in the body and dependencies on the drug.

Vaccines – Next time you are considering getting a vaccine, ask for the ingredients label first. You will notice nasty ingredients on this list including formaldehyde (a known carcinogen), fetal DNA, food proteins, and other questionable ingredients. This may make you question inserting them directly into your blood stream where your body can't filter through and process out the bad ingredients first. I know there is a lot of controversy surrounding this topic, but speaking from personal experience, vaccines can cause adverse reactions in your immune system. When these ingredients are put into your blood stream, your body not only attacks the virus but all the other ingredients (like food proteins), and this can cause your body to continue attacking those foods every time you eat them. A common example is eggs are used to create the flu vaccine, so naturally your body will attack the egg proteins when receiving the vaccine and continue doing so anytime you consume eggs.

Dehydration – When your body isn't getting enough water, the toxin riddled food that should be flushed out sits in your intestines, causing constipation. This allows the toxins that would normally be disposed to cause inflammation and pass through your intestines and into your blood stream.

Stress – This can cause your body to not produce the necessary hormones for correct digestive function. Stress also prevents your "happy hormone," serotonin, from being released into your blood stream, which causes more stress. It's a downward cycle. Many people might not believe that being stressed can affect your healing process, but it makes a major difference.

Why Avoiding the Foods That Make You Sick Isn't Enough

When your body becomes allergic to a certain food, you stop eating that food, and obviously you stop experiencing the pains caused by that allergy. Many people attempt to adjust their life around that. It works for a while, but then they start to get sick again.

This happens because the food that you eat (usually the food that you eat the most, but not always) continues to seep through your semi-permeable intestinal wall and more antibodies are created to purge that food. Now you are allergic to two food items, not just one. Obviously you see the major problem that comes from this, as eventually, you will be forced to adjust your diet again and again until there is nothing left for you to eat. I call this the "Degenerative Food Sensitivity Cycle."

Common symptoms

The degenerative food sensitivity cycle isn't the only problem that comes from these antigens seeping into your bloodstream. Your body can't get rid of every toxin that enters through your intestinal wall, and as these toxins build up over time, the ones that are not purged from your system will be absorbed by organs, muscles, joints and bones in your body.

Every part of your body can and will absorb some of these toxins. The more toxins that are put into your body, the more toxins your organs absorb, causing them (against their hardest efforts) to malfunction.

Since every part of your body depends on your blood stream to operate, every part of your body can be affected by Leaky Gut Syndrome, which essentially means any problem can be caused by Leaky Gut. This is one of the major reasons why the effects of Leaky Gut Syndrome are so diverse and difficult to diagnose.

Here is a list of some of the results that may come from toxins building up. Remember, this is in no way a complete list:

Food Allergies
Food Intolerances
Fatigue
Asthma
Ulcerative Colitis
Rheumatoid Arthritis
Depression
Anxiety

Irritable Bowel Syndrome
Celiac Disease
Ulcers
Acid reflux
Gall Bladder Disease
Burst Appendix
Multiple Sclerosis
Crohn's Disease
Anemia
Constipation
Fibromyalgia
Endometriosis
Lack of Mental Clarity
ADD/ADHD
Brain Fog
Dizziness
Stomach/Intestinal cramps
Irregular Periods
Menstrual Cramping
Excessive Gas
Loss of Appetite
Fevers
Passing Out
Sleeping Constantly
Light Headedness
Weak Muscles
UTI's and Bladder Problems
Body Aches
Bronchitis
Joint Pain
Shortness of Breath
Hiatal Hernia
Headaches
Migraines
Bad Memory
Bad Vision
Hot and Cold Flashes
Back Pain
Frequent Urination
Constant Hunger Pains
Hives
Flushing
Thrush

Hormonal Imbalances
Acne
Decrease in Immunity
POTS
Bi-Polar Disorder

These are only some of the problems that root from Leaky Gut Syndrome. Of course, Leaky Gut Syndrome is not the only cause of all of these problems but they all occur because of it.

Bad Immunity

When your body is so focused on getting rid of toxins, it fails to make as many defenses as it should and strengthen your immune system against other illnesses, leaving your body prone to more illness. It is not unusual if your body is constantly getting sick with the latest cold or flu.

Hormonal Imbalances

One last thing this can do to your body is create a hormonal imbalance. Your digestive system is responsible for releasing Serotonin, the "happy hormone," your body naturally produces. When your digestive system is weakened, it causes less Serotonin to be released. This can cause depression, anxiety, mood swings, bi-polar disorder and many other emotional problems. You can read more on that in chapter eight.

Other hormones are also affected which can cause any of your glands to malfunction or other hormonal problems.

What to Do

Remember that these problems are really only the offspring of one parent issue. Hospitals and doctors often treat these side effects as if they were individual problems, but in reality, *they are just side effects of one larger problem,* and by treating the side effects the way they do, they make the actual problem worse. This is called "Symptom Suppression." Whether medical science is ignorant of this, or the hospitals do it on purpose to ensure that you come back and spend more money, I don't know. All I know is that doctors don't usually diagnose leaky gut (unless you're lucky). They instead treat your numerous symptoms as individual problems with even more pills and medication. This of course adds to the original problem making your symptoms worse. Are you beginning to understand why symptom suppression doesn't work?

The best hope doctors often will offer you is to tell you that you have numerous health issues that will likely never get better and your only hope is that if they perform a surgery, or give a monumental effort, it won't get worse. Naturally, this isn't always true or I wouldn't be writing this book.

You see, our bodies were created to heal themselves. They know what to do if we allow them to do it. They know what their natural state is supposed to be, and if we allow them to heal, they will. The tricky part is giving our body the opportunity to get better. It needs to have the perfect environment to heal, and we can give it that.

2 DIAGNOSING LEAKY GUT

There are many ways to diagnose leaky gut. Often times, people will have so many of the symptoms that they just assume that they have it. Usually they are right.

*Note: I do recommend making a list of all of your symptoms. It's helpful to have this list during the healing process to see your progress.

Others need more reassurance. Some of the common tests people take are:

Intestinal Permeability Test
Blood Test for Antigens (IgE levels)
Skin Prick Allergy Test

These tests can be done by a local health-care practitioner.

I personally recommend getting a blood test because this seems to be more accurate than a skin prick test (remember, it's your blood that's attacking the antigens, not your skin). A skin prick test can be accurate too, but a blood test is usually more accurate.

This lets you know exactly what foods your body attacks and how bad your reactions are. It also tells you which foods are passing through your intestinal wall into your blood stream since it is testing the antigens in your blood.

There are also intestinal permeability home test kits available at Lab Testing Direct or Accesa Labs. These directly test for Leaky Gut Syndrome and have proven to be very useful. You can order them online.

Process of Elimination

Another thing people do is eliminate one food at a time (or reintroduce them one at a time if they are already on a strict diet) in order to see which ones they react to. This works well when you are unsure what foods make you sick and which ones do not, but it can be complicated to find a control in this experiment. You must be sure to document your eating habits and symptoms in a food journal. Doing so will make this process easier.

Muscle Testing

Another way to find out what foods you react to is through muscle testing. This is a controversial method since many people don't believe the chemistry behind it works, but it is very commonly benefited from and free, so there's no harm in trying. There are many YouTube videos that are very good at demonstrating how to perform muscle testing at home and explaining how it works. There are also holistic doctors who practice muscle testing that you can look into.

*Tests are not always accurate

I wanted to mention that sometimes specific problems won't show up on tests even if you do have them. This has a lot to do with your blood chemistry, what you've eaten recently, and many other factors. If you feel like you have leaky gut but don't test positive for it, please take heart. You can still follow the guidelines in this book and get your life back. This is something anyone can do and benefit greatly from.

3 HOW TO HEAL NATURALLY

Many people hope for a miracle pill or something that will get rid of their leaky gut for them. Honestly, that may be why you have this problem in the first place. If you have a health issue and you take it to the doctor looking for the "miracle pill" the doctor will be happy to acquiesce and will prescribe you some pills. As you have probably figured out now, those pills can cause you all of the problems that you're trying to avoid.

Medication can be life-saving in some instances, but I don't believe that we should rely on them to "fix" everything (the word fix is in quotation marks because medication does not, never has and never will fix anything. It simply suppresses unpleasant symptoms).

*Note: I understand there are cases where medication is necessary to stay alive. These are the exceptions, not the rule.

Our bodies were never meant to rely on medication, and since we can't go more than a few days without food, wouldn't it make sense that that basic necessity would be exactly what we need to heal our bodies? People are always chasing after the next miracle pill and expensive medication, when in reality, the best "medication" we can offer our bodies is a steady solid diet every single day. It's really that simple.

Let me put it this way, if you can't find the time or money to eat right and exercise now, you'll have to find the time and money to visit the doctor and have numerous health issues later.

Be Patient

At this point you're probably thinking, "Yeah, it would be nice to get better and this is certainly interesting, but why can't you just tell me how to start healing?" I will! Don't worry about that yet. My point in telling you this is so you understand that this isn't a miracle pill. It does take time and dedication and can be very taxing, but if you give it a chance and work hard to give your body what it needs, you will get better.

Why You Should Heal Naturally

Now one more thing before we get started. I want you to understand why I am writing about healing naturally. There isn't a miracle pill that you can take that will "solve" all of your health problems (remember why the word fix was in quotation marks a few paragraphs ago? Yeah, same reason). For example, when you break a bone in your arm, do you take a pill every day and call it good by using your arm just as you would any other day? Or do you have surgery to take the bone out and just live without it for the rest of your life? I sincerely hope you answered no to those questions. Why would you not do that? Because it doesn't work.

It's common sense that with a broken bone you put it in a cast and allow it to heal naturally. You take care of it and allow it to get better on its own. Believe it or not, your organs are the exact same way (aside from putting them in a cast). Sometimes our bodies are damaged and we need to let them repair before using them normally again. That's how we heal leaky gut: *naturally and with time* (How much time? We'll get into that later, but for now don't panic).

Who is it For?

This isn't for everybody. It takes time, dedication and work but if you are willing to do that, your benefits will be great. Understand that this is not simply a change of diet that you will undergo, it is a lifestyle change. It's not easy, but it will help you get your life back on track. Not everybody has the same work ethic (yes, this requires some work) but this is not the project in the back yard that you can get halfway through and give up until next spring. If you're not serious about healing, don't even bother.

What You Should Eat and Why

I know many people focus on what they can't eat while eating healthy, but understand that with what we do, that kind of negative mindset is dangerous. It's more likely to make you give up than anything else. Bearing that in mind, I am going to start with what you can have. Let me just say that there is SO much you can eat while healing your gut. A lot of it is being creative and figuring out how to cook, especially if you don't know how, but I will teach you everything I know. It's always best to look on the bright side.

Water

I can't stress this point enough. You need to drink water. You are supposed to drink 1/2 your body weight in ounces every day, so if you weigh 150 pounds, you would need to drink 75 ounces of water per day. Do you? Probably not. Start being conscientious of how much water you drink. It's important.

Now let me stress that drinking water is one of the most overlooked aspects of healing your leaky gut. Think about it. You have all of those toxins flowing through your body and in order to flush those toxins out your body needs extra water.

Drinking enough and even extra water gives your body the ability to flush out the toxins faster than it would when you don't get enough water, which allows you to heal faster.

You know when you have a cold and you feel like you are running to the bathroom every few minutes, even though you're not drinking that much? Your body is flushing out all of the toxins so you will get over your cold faster. It is the same concept with Leaky Gut.

Lack of water is also one of the biggest causes of constipation and headaches. Drink water and you will feel better.

Another tip to drinking enough water is to carry a water bottle around with you (I think buying a really awesome one helps). When you have it in front of you, you are more likely to drink, and in turn, more likely to feel better sooner.

Juice and Other Fluids

Another note is that many people think they can drink other fluids instead of water. If you do want to drink another fluid you can drink 100% fresh squeezed fruit juice, but only moderately. You shouldn't drink more than a glass a day. You can also use unsweetened coconut milk. This should be used moderately. Fruit juice is not bad for you, but the kind of juice that you buy in the store (even if it says 100% juice) has concentrated fruit sugars that your body can't process. None of that is good for you.

*If you are craving juice, try V8, the completely vegetable kind with no added ingredients (Yes, I know that tomato is a fruit but I include it when I say "completely vegetable." Bring it up with the creator of V8). It's really tasty and good for you, even though it's "technically" V7-F1.

Protein

Protein is very important in rebuilding muscle, organs and body functions. You should eat protein with every meal.

Meat

Meat is so important in healing your body. It has so many nutrients and is very good for your body; however, you should not eat pork since it is high in salt and fat content and really not that great for healing. You can eat:

    Chicken
    Turkey
    Beef (has most nutrients)
    Lamb
    Fish (great for omega 3)
    NO Pork
    Others

Eggs

Eggs are very good for you, and can be eaten daily (just make sure you're not allergic to them first), but they should not be used as a replacement for meat. You need meat in order to heal, but eggs are a good healthy source of protein as well.

    *Eggs are a great source of protein for breakfast.

Nuts

Nuts, if you do not react to them, are good for you to eat moderately. They should not be used as a replacement for your protein intake. Nuts are a good addition to your diet but are not necessary for healing. Sadly, you should not eat peanuts. They are one of the easiest things to become allergic to. Now let's take a look at the bright side. Some of the nuts you can have are:

    Cashews
    Almonds
    Pecans
    Walnuts
    Hazelnuts
    Pistachios
    Chestnuts
    Pinenuts
    NO Peanuts

You can also eat seeds. These include:
    Sunflower seeds

Pumpkins seeds

Fruit

Some people might say to avoid fruit while healing Leaky Gut because it can feed candida (which is discussed later) because it contains fructose (natural fruit sugar). Actually, fruit is mandatory for healing Leaky Gut. Fruit does contain natural fruit sugar, but it is not refined or processed and is actually necessary for keeping your blood sugar balanced while healing your body. Fruit should be eaten consistently. For example, while I was healing I would eat 5-7 peaches, apples, oranges, or other fruit per day. The only fruit you shouldn't eat is bananas. They are hard to digest and can cause constipation. Some of the fruits you can eat are:

Apples
Strawberries
Blueberries
Blackberries
Raspberries
Oranges
Lemons
Limes
Grapefruit
Mango
Kiwi
Peaches
Nectarines
Grapes
Pears
Other
NO Bananas

Vegetables

Vegetables are very important in healing your gut. They contain many of the necessary tools to rebuild your body and will give you fiber which helps with constipation. You should eat vegetables with every meal. You should not eat potatoes because of the starch. Many people also avoid nightshades, though I only recommend doing so if you feel better without them.

You should also avoid corn because it has no nutrients and turns into sugar. You can eat tomatoes, onions and garlic (which is essential for healing) every day but you should rotate the rest of your vegetables. Some of the vegetables you can eat are:

Onions
Tomatoes
Avocados
Garlic
Asparagus
Zucchini
Spaghetti Squash
Sweet Potatoes
Acorn Squash
Green Beans
Peas
Mushrooms
Carrots
Bell Peppers
Cucumber
Beets
Spinach
Others
NO Potatoes
NO Corn
NO Iceberg Lettuce

If you find that certain vegetables do not make you feel well, try cooking them in a little bit of water or oil over the stove. The chemical composition of food changes when it's cooked and many people find that they react to uncooked fruits and vegetables but not to cooked ones.

Either way, you should always cook your vegetables in a little bit of water or oil over the stove. This helps keep the nutrients in one place while changing the composition of the vegetable into something more easily digested.

Herbs and Seasonings

Herbs are very good for you and should be used for healing. Seasonings should not have extra ingredients in them and should only be natural. A good rule is if you don't know what everything is in a label, you shouldn't eat it. Some common herbs and seasonings you can use are:

Rock Salt
Pepper
Garlic Powder
Onion Powder

Oregano (great for healing so use liberally)
Cilantro
Parsley
Chives
Cracked Peppercorn
Basil
Rosemary
Thyme
Sage

Oils and Butter

Vegetable oils should not be used for cooking. They are saturated fats and do not aid in healing. You can use olive oil, coconut oil and organic 100% butter interchangeably.

Other Foods to Include

Other foods that are imperative for healing are:

Bone Broth: one of the cheapest most beneficial foods to include in your healing. It has a lot of calcium and magnesium as well as gelatin which is high in inflammatory amino-acids.

Honey: Great for healing and contains all of the essential enzymes for living. As a bonus it also helps with seasonal allergies and blood-sugar. It's documented that honey doesn't feed Candida, although it should still be used moderately.

Apple Cider Vinegar: contains many amino acids and enzymes that aid in healing and digestion

100% Cocoa: increases blood flow, balances cholesterol, high in antioxidants and magnesium

Cod Liver Oil: contains more Vitamin A and D than any other natural food and contains many minerals that strengthen the intestines. Whether in pill form or liquid, it's very good for you. Be sure to buy one that's fermented and non-toxic. I recommend the Green Pasture brand.

Cinnamon: reduces inflammations, contains anti-oxidants and fights bacteria

Coconut Oil: fights off yeast and fungus, regulates blood sugar, increases metabolism and thyroid function

Oregano: helps moderate candida, contains fiber, iron, magnesium, calcium, vitamin E, vitamin K, Omega-3's and antioxidants

Garlic: anti-parasitic, bacterial and fungal, contains many antioxidants.

Things To Note

Although it might make you sad, you will probably be making most things from scratch. You should not be eating processed foods that come in cans, boxes, bags, or other packaging (no almond flour or that type of stuff). These foods almost always contain preservatives, chemicals and hormones. You are not eating junk food, so you can expect to make most things from scratch.

Note: Some people may have adverse reactions to specific vegetables, fruits, meats, etc. ***You should alter your diet accordingly and eat what makes YOU feel best.*** We are all different, so naturally your diet will be different than mine.

What You Shouldn't Eat and Why

While this section is important, I don't want it to be the focus of your next few months simply because I want you to have your mind focused on what you can have and that you are giving your body what it needs. However, I do need to talk about the different things you shouldn't be eating in order to help you understand and be okay with not eating these foods.

No Sugar

One of the hardest things for most people to stop eating is sugar. Most people are addicted to it without even knowing it. Sugar is a poison that our bodies have adapted to because we eat it so often, but it causes problems. Not only does it make us chronically tired, but it converts straight into fat and also causes many of our bodily functions to go awry.

When you have sugar withdrawals, your energy levels drop and your symptoms flare. This is because, like any other drug or poison, our bodies can become addicted to it, and it happens all the time. This is where those sugar cravings come from.

As soon as you stop eating sugar and give your body time to adjust, you will feel a drastic change in your energy levels, but don't expect to get over it instantly. You're going to experience some withdrawals. My suggestion is to keep some frozen grapes near at hand so you can conquer that sweet tooth whenever you get a craving. It works better than you would expect and is super tasty.

Unfortunately, not eating sugar isn't enough. You must also not eat any sugar replacements including: High Fructose Corn Syrup, Corn Syrup, Stevia, Aspartame, Splenda, Agave Nectar or any other artificial sugar replacer.

To prevent sugar cravings and balance blood sugar, you need to eat a good amount of fruit every day, and you can have honey moderately. This will give your body what it needs without allowing it to succumb to those sugar cravings and withdrawals.

*Make sure the honey you get is 100% raw honey. Most of the hone sold in stores has corn syrup added. Try a small local market or farm for the best honey. Eating local honey also helps with local seasonal allergies.

No Grains

This is another one of those hard things to give up, especially since it is the main staple in today's society. There are two different types of grains I want to talk about. The first is refined grains, the other is whole grains.

Grains are made up of three components: the bran (outer layer), endosperm (middle layer), and the germ (inner layer). The bran and germ are the most nutritious parts of the grain and contain almost all of the fiber, minerals, vitamins and antioxidants. When a grain is refined, those two parts are removed and all that is left is the endosperm which is mostly starchy carbohydrates with little to no nutrients. These carbohydrates convert to sugar in your body and are usually stored as fat or disposed. Because of this, when you are eating refined grains you are eating empty calories and not doing anything beneficial to your body. That means no white bread. It should even be avoided after you heal your body. Corn should be avoided as it has little to no nutritional value and is an empty food source. It is considered a grain in this diet and should not be eaten.

*Tip: If you are feeling very hungry without carbs, try eating sweet potatoes, squash, or avocados. These are all filling and will help your body get the carbs it needs. It may take a while for your body to get used to not eating grains, and you may feel hungry at first, but don't be afraid to try new foods and eat the things that make you feel good. And especially don't be afraid to eat enough. It's really hard to gain weight eating this way, so eat until you're full.

Whole Grains

I want to emphasize that whole grains are very good for you. Wheat especially is the staple of life and brings a lot of value into your diet. Now with that being said, whole grains are very hard to digest. Most healthy bodies can handle that and have strong enough stomachs to break up grains and digest them, and this actually adds to their value, but when you have leaky gut your body needs the most stress-free and ideal environment to heal.

In order to rebuild your digestive system, you must have an easy diet for your body to process, and often times that includes refraining from all grains.

Wheat is also one of the most common reactants and should also be avoided for that reason.

Once your body is healed and your stomach stronger, whole grains are a great way to keep your body healthy and strong. We will talk more about what to do after you are healed later.

No Dairy

Dairy is hard on your digestive system which is not good for a body that needs to get better. It is a common cause of constipation, diarrhea and cramps when you are sick, and is also one of the most common intolerances that people have.

Another problem with dairy is the amount of hormones and antibiotics put into it in today's world. Remember how antibiotics are one of the biggest causes of leaky gut? Those antibiotics are in our milk and do not help with healing or restoring the digestive system.

100% Organic Butter is allowed on this protocol because the chemical composition of it is different than milk and other dairy products. You may also try organic goat milk and cheese or raw organic cow milk with **NO** additives *if* you do not react to it. These should be eaten sparingly and should not be eaten with any sign of a reaction.

No Soy

Soy is another one of those over-processed foods that is not good for you. The soy used in our food today contains a component that mimics estrogen, as well as other things that are not good for you. Soybean in its original form is generally okay for you in moderation, but while you are healing any form of soy is not recommended.

No Peanuts

Peanuts should be abstained from because they are one of the most common allergies. This indicates that they are easier to become allergic to than most foods. They also contain aflatoxins which are naturally occurring fungal toxins which is obviously not beneficial to your body. Because of this you should not eat peanuts in any form, regardless of whether you react to them or not.

No Vegetable or Canola Oils

You should not use vegetable oils. Like many refined things, vegetable oil, canola oil and shortening are derived from food that has had all of the nutrients sapped out. They also contain fats that are not beneficial to your body. Many may tell you otherwise, but the bottom line is these are not good for you and should not be used, especially while healing your body. You will feel much better and healthier using olive oil, butter and coconut oil.

NO Caffeine

If you love your coffee, trying heating up some coconut milk on the stove and adding 100% cocoa and honey to it instead. You can also try various herbal teas. Caffeine is a stimulant and wears out your body, as well as causes your body to become reliant on it.

Others

NO Pork
NO Potatoes
NO Bananas
NO Coffee
NO Tea that isn't herbal
NO Alcohol or Drugs
NO Corn
NO Legumes
NO Processed, Boxed, or Canned Foods
NO Almond flours, artificial sweeteners, etc.

Some Notes

This eating plan will reduce inflammation in the gut and provide the perfect environment for healing. Because of the nature of the eating plan I am presenting, you should plan on making most all of the foods you eat from scratch. Whole foods simply aren't sold in most groceries stores pre-cooked without preservatives, un-wanted seasonings, marinades, sauces, etc. You are not eating junk food and should be expecting to cook.

 I know it is hard to take time and find the motivation to cook, but many find that after they start cooking all of their meals and start feeling well again, they actually gain time because they have more energy, can manage things better, and can get more things done in smaller amounts of time. It may be hard at first but it is most definitely worth it.

 It will be hard and take much time and dedication, but it will be the most rewarding thing you can do for yourself, especially right now.

4 IMPORTANT CONCEPTS

Food Journal

First of all, it is very helpful to keep a food journal. This includes writing down everything you eat organized by meal/day. Keeping a food journal helps you pin point foods that you react to and it also helps you more easily rotate your foods which we will talk about next. I recommending finding a food journal you're motivated to write in, whether it be a journal, notebook, word processor document, or app (some apps even let you take pictures of all your meals).

Food Rotation

A very important and commonly overlooked factor in healing leaky gut is rotating your foods. You should eat a certain type of food in one 24-hour time period, and then you shouldn't eat that food again for three days, meaning you have a four-day food rotation. You only eat the same foods every four days.

    For example, on Sunday I may eat beef and asparagus for dinner. I would then eat my left-overs for lunch the next day. Then I wouldn't eat beef or asparagus for another three day period, or until Thursday night for dinner. I usually eat my dinner left-overs for lunch the next day. You don't have to eat the same foods in the same day, just in the same 24-hour time period. That way you can have a variety of foods each day.

    By rotating your foods, you are preventing yourself from creating new reactions to foods. This is how we avoid the Degenerative Food Sensitivity

Cycle.

Another good thing about rotating foods is that you can pin-point your exact food reactions. If you feel great every day except for the days you eat chicken, you know which food is making you sick.

Below there is a sample of my food journal combined with a food rotation sample when I was healing my leaky gut.

Food Rotation Chart

Day 1	Day 2	Day 3	Day 4
Breakfast: Strawberries Blueberries	**Breakfast** Peaches Mango	**Breakfast** Eggs Bell Peppers Coconut Milk Cocoa Powder	**Breakfast** Raspberries Blackberries Almond Milk
Lunch Sweet Potatoes Onions Mushrooms Beef	**Lunch** Oranges Chicken Asparagus Honey	**Lunch** Bell Peppers Turkey Grapes	**Lunch** Salmon Lettuce Tomatoes
Snacks Almonds Pears	**Snacks** Apples Cocoa Powder Hazelnuts Honey	**Snacks** Zuchinni Cashews	**Snacks** Green Beans Kiwis
Dinner Oranges Chicken Asparagus Honey	**Dinner** Bell Peppers Turkey Acorn Squash	**Dinner** Salmon Lettuce Tomatoes	**Dinner** Spaghetti Squash Tomato Sauce Ground Beef

No Microwave

I know, it sounds crazy, but this really is important. When you microwave food, the waves that penetrate your food and heat it up actually magnify and multiply the toxins in your food as well as kill off many of the important nutrients your body needs. That's why when you heat up breastmilk for a baby, you do so over the stove. Because of this it is best not to use a microwave for heating up or cooking food. Toaster-ovens or a regular oven, as well as a pan or pot are great alternatives and keep the nutrients in your food. I recommend toaster ovens as they are inexpensive to buy and operate, and they heat up food much faster than a regular oven. As an added bonus, it also makes your food crispy and tasty. I also use stainless steel pots and pans as well as cast iron to cook over the stove. Having good cooking utensils makes cooking more enjoyable and much easier.

Meal Proportions

I wanted to talk a little bit about meal proportions. Many people recommend eating specific amounts of food every meal. My mind honestly gets overwhelmed thinking that way and I prefer working in much simpler ways. Realize that our bodies will naturally crave the foods they need, and it is also just extra stress trying to integrate another thing into your life.

I would just recommend trying to keep your meals as balanced as possible, meaning, take care to eat protein and carbohydrates in a balanced manner.

Something I would recommend is eating **five small meals every day** and snacking in-between those meals. This keeps your metabolism going and allows your body to thoroughly use the food you are feeding it. I also have seen that most people feel better after implementing this principle.

Remember, this habits may seem small but it's the small things that make a world of difference when you're working toward getting better.

5 SLEEP, EXERCISE AND REDUCING STRESS

There are many factors that deal directly with healing and how well you heal. The most important things are food and supplements, but there other important factors you will need that will aid you in healing Leaky Gut.

Sleep

Something that society today really has a hard time with is taking time to sleep. Our world is so busy that we believe we can't take time for ourselves, not even time to take care of ourselves. If you are in this mindset, look at it this way. If we take a little time for ourselves now, we will be able to have a lot more time in the future to do everything we need to accomplish. This includes taking time to sleep.

We heal the most while we sleep, especially when we are getting at least 8 hours of sleep a night. We also get better rest when we go to sleep earlier at night and get up earlier in morning, sleeping when the sun does and waking up with it. There's much truth to the old saying, "Early to bed, early to rise, makes a man healthy, wealthy and wise." While being wealthy and wise would be nice, let's just try and focus on being healthy for now.

The best time for rest is between 10:30PM and 6AM. I know with our busy lives it's hard to get to bed at such a decent (or crazy, depending on your current schedule) hour, but if you at least try to get in bed earlier you will notice a big change in how you feel or at least in your productivity. Getting enough sleep will also help you heal faster which will give you more time and a better life. Taking time to heal your body now keeps you healthier in the long run.

Exercise

Another important factor in this healthy lifestyle is exercise. Exercising helps build muscle and dispose of toxins. It also stimulates the release of serotonin and helps provide energy. There are so many benefits to exercising and different kinds of exercise offer different benefits. I would suggest avoiding especially stressful forms of exercise like running, but my advice is to find a form of exercise you enjoy and sticking with it. It doesn't so much matter *what* you do so long as you're doing *something.*

A lot of people enjoy yoga which is a very good form of exercise (and meditation, more on that later) and which is good for healing. My favorite yoga videos are done by Erin Motz in Do You Yoga's 30-Day Yoga Challenge. Yoga is a great way to release stress, relax the body, and build muscle all at the same time.

Zumba is also great exercise for those who can exert more. Even simply stretching or speed walking, or walking at all are good starts for getting back on track to a healthy lifestyle.

While I was healing, I ballroom danced every day. Every morning it was hard to gather the necessary energy and motivation, but once there I would somehow find the energy I needed. If I wasn't able to go, I would turn on music and dance with my roommates. This was something I loved and enjoyed, and it provided me with a form of exercise. So I'll say again that it doesn't so much matter what you're doing, so long as you're doing something.

In light of this, if you want a quick laugh, Google "Prancercise." This is a perfect example of finding something that you enjoy doing that works for you.

Meditation

Back to meditation; there is something healing about focusing on your breathing and calming your mind that helps you relax and simply feel better. I recommend finding a quiet place every day for just a few minutes to focus only on your breathing and let the rest of your stresses and problems leave for a while.

Meditation helps relieve stress and tension and can keep you motivated to heal your Leaky Gut. Even if you're not the "meditating type," you should try it.

Reduce Stress

One last thing you should focus on is reducing stress and eliminating unnecessary stresses. I know this is easier said than done, but think about the things in your life and see if there is any way to reduce the amount of stress they give you or even a way you can take a break from those things for now.

If you cannot change them, focus your mind on not letting them stress you out. The things we can't change we should work on being okay with and not let them lower our spirits. Stress not only makes things harder than they should be. It aggravates the inflammation in your body, so make an effort to reduce stress in your life.

On that note, if there is something specific I have suggested doing that just causes you stress to even think about doing, take a deep breath and don't worry about implementing that thing right now. If the times comes in the future and you want to try it, great, but stress has such a negative impact on your body that trying to fit something in and being stressed about it is actually worse than forgetting that initial step all together.

Other Things to Do

Salt baths: These help release toxins in the body and reduce inflammation.

Hot showers/baths: These increase blood flow and help release toxins.

Massages: These increase blood flow and releases toxins from muscles. Be sure to drink lots of fluid before and after so the toxins that are released from the muscles get flushed out. We use a mini massager (that we love!).

Stretching: This builds strength and helps release toxins in muscles. It also releases endorphins that make you happy and give you energy.

6 SUPPLEMENTS

Note: You should work with a health care practitioner when considering taking these supplements. The last thing you want to do is throw your body off because there was not a proper knowledge of the supplements and their effects on your body beforehand. As stated before, the information in this book is only meant to supplement, not replace, your health care practitioner's knowledge and work, and should only be used in conjunction with them.

I cannot stress how important these supplements are to healing your body. It is common for those who eat on the previously outlined diet to feel better, even if they don't take the supplements, but when they try to reintroduce the foods they were allergic to into their diets, they learn that they still have the same food sensitivities. That is what most people consider healing, but I don't believe you are completely healed until you are completely free from all pain and health problems, and you can attain this. I know because I've done it, and I've helped countless others do it too.

There are people who start taking supplements and actually start to feel worse, so they assume that the supplements won't work, when really, the sickness they feel comes from the massive buildup of toxins purging from their systems. When this is the case, it is recommended to stop taking the supplements and to continue eating on the previously outlined diet for a few more weeks until more toxins have had a chance to leave your system.

You should not start the supplements until you have properly purged your body of many toxins and are consistently eating on the diet outlined in the previous chapter, which usually takes about 4-8 weeks.

These supplements not only help get rid of all of your symptoms but they rebuild your digestive system and body, and allow you to live a normal lifestyle again without having to worry about eating something that may send you to your death bed.

That's what the supplements are for. They kick your body into overdrive and turn your organs into healing power houses.

That being said, it is perfectly acceptable to eat on the previously outlined diet and not worry about supplements. It may take you longer to heal, but your body will feel better than it ever has.

L-Glutamine

Many amino acids can be used for rebuilding your digestive tract, but one of the most common is L-Glutamine. This amino acid helps build and strengthen the intestines while also supplying essential components for rebuilding muscle.

There are many different types of L-Glutamine and some are better quality than others. I would recommend doing your research before purchasing any one brand. Your health care practitioner may also have a brand they recommend that you cannot get over the counter. These are usually higher quality and what I would recommend going with, as with all the supplements. You won't want to start taking L-Glutamine until you feel your body is ready to start rebuilding itself and you are done with the toxin purging phase, usually at least a month or two after starting the other supplements. This is because L-Glutamine rebuilds your digestive system and you can't rebuild it until all of the inflammation is gone.

Probiotics/Prebiotics

One of the biggest problems with having leaky gut is the imbalance of bacteria in the digestive system, especially when you have candida or have taken antibiotics. Probiotics replace the missing beneficial bacteria and balance the gut. Anytime you take antibiotics you should take probiotics as well. They should be taken while healing leaky gut to help restore the missing bacteria.

As with all of the supplements, I recommend doing your research for brands. Find one that is quality with quality ingredients and no extra unnecessary additives.

Enzymes

When your body is focused on getting rid of toxins and handling stress, it doesn't always focus on providing imperative enzymes for healing. These include liver, pancreatic and digestive enzymes. Without enough of these enzymes, your body becomes more stressed which in turn makes leaky gut worse. These supplements make the digestion process flow while giving your body the ability to focus on healing and repairing.

Digestive Herbs

There are many herbs that reduce inflammation in the gut and calm the digestive system to make repairs easier as well as boost the immune system and function. These are not always necessary but in severe cases can be *very* beneficial. They also speed up the healing process.

Magnesium

Constipation is a major problem with leaky gut. It not only stresses out the digestive system but allows more food to pass through your intestinal wall into your bloodstream. Apart from this it will make your life more comfortable. Magnesium is something you can take for constipation. It has many benefits but it can be used as a laxative if constipation is bad, especially while taking the other leaky gut supplements. This is something to only get if you need it, meaning it's optional but very useful.

There are many supplements you can take that will aid in healing, and most people talking about healing leaky gut will recommend a combination of these and possible a few others. I recommend using these supplements specifically because they are the ones I personally used to heal and have seen many others use to heal. I want to emphasize that you know your body the best and you should be knowledgeable about what you put into. Do your research on brands and find something that will work for you.

As for a protocol, I do recommend working with a health care practitioner because you are dealing with products that can have tremendous effects on your body, and everyone's body is different. If you would like direction, though, I recommend following a protocol like the one Dr. Josh Axe recommends. You can easily find it on his website, or feel free to contact me.

Remember, you can do this and you can get better.

7 CANDIDA

What is Candida?

I know I've mentioned candida a lot, and now you finally get to learn more about it. Candida refers to the overgrowth of the bacteria called "candida" that is naturally occurring in the digestive tract. Everybody has Candida in their digestive tract, so the real problem is not the actual presence of Candida; it's the overabundance of it. This is often caused by an imbalance in the digestive system which can be caused by many things. Some of the most common causes are:

Antibiotics
Poor Diet
Pathogenic Infection

When you take antibiotics, you wipe out ALL of the bacteria in your digestive tract, good and bad. As with all things, the bad grows and takes over much more quickly than the good, so when they are both wiped out, the bad bacteria grows unchecked and unbalanced. You might think that instead of taking antibiotics once and then letting the Candida take over you will continue to take antibiotics and just keep both down to solve the problem, but in reality If you take antibiotics often, candida will become immune to it and then completely take over. Obviously, this causes a lot of problems in the digestive tract.

Differences Between Leaky Gut and Candida
How They Make Each Other Worse

Leaky Gut and Candida are often times related but the two are entirely different issues. One of these sicknesses can exist without the other, although they can easily lead to the other and often do.

Candida refers to the overgrowth of a specific species of yeast within the digestive tract which, if left untreated, can and will continue to create intestinal inflammation that leads to Leaky Gut.

The opposite can be true as well. Having Leaky Gut can cause your digestive system to become a breeding ground for Candida.

When you have Candida Overgrowth and Leaky Gut, the Candida is allowed to pass through your intestinal wall into the blood stream. From there it can travel to any part of your body making Leaky Gut much worse. You can see how this problem is continually degenerative.

In whichever case, it's always related to the imbalance of gut flora within the digestive tract.

How to Know if You Have Candida

Most people realize they have Candida overgrowth when they have strong sugar cravings and withdrawals after they stop eating any form of sugar. Since sugar feeds Candida, eliminating sugar starves the Candida and causes die-off effects which include any of the symptoms you've been having among other things. When the Candida in your body is being starved, you may have many withdrawal symptoms as if your body were addicted to a drug. These symptoms can include:

Extreme Fatigue
Extreme Sugar Cravings
Shakiness
Diarrhea and Constipation
Light-headedness
Flushing
Thrush/White Colored Tongue
Chronic Yeast Infection
Dandruff
Gas, Burping and Bloating
Other variety of problems

This is very common and can be alleviated by keeping yourself hydrated, taking the recommended supplements, getting a lot of rest, eating some fruits and abstaining completely from sugar. When the Candida begins to die off, your effects will be much stronger and more painful than normal, but being persist and getting through it and it will make a major difference.

To test yourself for Candida Overgrowth, you can perform a saliva test, get tested by a holistic doctor, or take a survey online.

If You Have Candida

This part is important, so read carefully. Your intestinal tract cannot heal while infested with Candida. You have to rid your body of Candida overgrowth first before you can focus on healing Leaky Gut.

How to Heal Candida

Luckily there are some simple ways to heal candida. I would recommend eating on the previously outlined diet provided while implementing the information below.

Candida feeds off of any type of sugar including sugar found in grains so you should eliminate all sugar, grains, and sugar replacements. Many people try to eliminate all fruit and honey as well, but if you need to balance blood sugar, honey is easier to digest than any other sweet food and is less likely to feed Candida. Also, I wouldn't suggest eliminating all fruit. Instead, I would try to eliminate all except:

Green Apples
Grapefruit
Berries
Avocado
Lemons
Limes

If you are allergic to all of the fruit listed above, understand that eating fruit is better than eating grains or sugar, so if you need a bigger variety of food in your diet, you can add some low-sugar and low-starch fruits back in that are not included on the list.

I would also recommend avoiding all yeast products including mushrooms. These foods feed and encourage candida and should be eliminated while starving the bacteria (starving sounds mean, but it really is what we're doing).

To help starve Candida and balance your digestive bacteria function, you should use *oregano oil* or oregano in your daily diet.

Be wary that the die-off effects of Candida can be brutal. If you are finding your symptoms getting worse as you eliminate fruit, try coming back to this later or eliminating the fruit more slowly. Many people give up completely because they can't eliminate fruit, but you can and will get better even if you don't eliminate fruit. It simply takes longer, which is just fine. I never actually eliminated fruit from my diet. I just gave myself more time to heal which worked better for me.

8 DEPRESSION AND ANXIETY

Before I address these issues, I want to mention that while there are many cases that changing your diet and exercise routine to something better for you often does help depression and anxiety, these are not always caused by eating patterns or leaky gut. Depression and anxiety are very real and can be caused by many factors.

That being said, I have never seen a case where someone changed the way they ate and it didn't help them feel at least some relief from their symptoms. Not all depression and anxiety is caused by nutrition problems, but it usually can be helped through eating right.

How it Works

Feeling depressed and anxious alongside leaky gut is completely normal. Your body's natural happy hormone, serotonin, is produced in the gut, and when something else is occupying the gut's concentration, like leaky gut, digestive issues, allergies, or other problems, producing that happy hormone is the first thing to get put aside. Without that happy hormone being produced, you are more prone to feeling depressed and anxious.

Reviving Our Body's Production of Serotonin

Like all problems, there is a cause. Since this type of depression and anxiety is caused by digestive problems and issues in the gut, it would only make sense to fix those digestive issues in order to get the body to generate serotonin again. By eating right, you can create a perfect environment for your body to heal, which also in turn allows your body to take up its normal functions like producing serotonin regularly.

There is also a flip side to this. Most people think they eat well, but don't realize how much stress they are putting on their gut. Even after healing their gut, many people eat food that is hard on the digestive system, and even a little bit of stress on the digestive system can inhibit some production of serotonin. It would make sense that when we eat better, more serotonin is produced, and we are happier.

Ideally, eating a perfect diet would make us perfectly happy. Of course, life is hard and things don't always go our way, but we would be happy more.

Even if eating a balanced, healthy diet seems hard, it's the best thing you can do for yourself and your body.

It's worth every bite.

Natural Remedies

There are a few natural remedies I would recommend looking into that are also known to help aid these issues.

Chamomile Herbal Tea

Chamomile's known effect on the body is to help it relax. It has also been used for hundreds of years as a natural remedy for anxiety.

Essential Oils

There are many benefits to essential oils, and one of the known benefits is help with relaxing the body and mind. The oils I'd look into are Lavender and Orange

Getting Out

Try getting out of the house and into nature. One of the best places to clear your mind and allow stress and anxiety to leave are in nature (mountains, beach, etc).

Although these are basic things, often they make a world of difference. If these don't help, healing Leaky Gut can eradicate or at least lesson depression. If these do not help and healing does not help, *do not be discouraged*. Often the greatest minds are those that feel emotions the deepest, and those who are prone to depression. Talk to someone. I have a Facebook group full of people going through healing leaky gut, and you might just find a friend. Send me a request to join that group here: https://www.facebook.com/groups/leakygut/

9 LIVING AFTER LEAKY GUT

It's a strange feeling to go from having so many health problems and eating restrictions to being able to eat whatever you'd like. There is a definite balance of eating well and enjoying what you eat. Here are a few tricks and tips to keep you healthy and leaky gut free.

Stay away from processed grains. These are empty calories and will only add fat to your body. These are also addicting and convert straight to sugar.

Eat whole grains if you want to eat grains. These will work your digestive system and make it stronger since whole grains are harder to break down. They also build up your body and keep you healthy.

Avoid any form of processed or unnatural sugar. Regardless of how yummy it tastes, sugar is never good for you and your body will attack it or become addicted to it if you're not careful. Other foods will become sweeter as you avoid sugar too, so it's easily worth it. It's easiest to stay away from sugar once you stop eating it. You will feel better and will avoid many health problems in the future. That isn't a requirement, but it is highly suggested. Avoiding sugar does not include avoiding fruit, honey, or other natural and unprocessed forms of fruit. These are good and healthy for you.

Stay away from processed food. Processed foods contain chemicals, hormones and preservatives that will bring additional health problems in the future and disrupt the balance of your body. Make your food homemade and whole whenever you can.

Obviously, when you finish this, you can eat however you like, and shouldn't be expected to stay on the diet the rest of your life, but a good suggestion for most people is to eat 80/20, meaning 80% of the time you eat on the foods previously outlined and 20% you can fluctuate. Be careful to think about how little 20% is because it will easily become more than that if you don't keep it in check. You will feel better eating well so I suggest that you do. A good rule is to eat natural foods. If they're natural and whole, you're likely getting a good balance while eating the rights foods.

If you start feeling more tired than usual or start seeing your old symptoms come back, this is usually caused by bad diet, medication, or other external factors. If you eat right, you shouldn't have any more major problems with your health, but it's best to take care to treat your body. It deserves to eat well and so do you.

Don't go back to eating how you were eating before.

The worst thing you can do for your body is go back to your old habits. You just made new ones and your body is thriving from this new way of living. If you continue to take care of your body, you will stay healthy. If you go back to your old eating habits, it's not uncommon to bring back many of your old health problems. Take care of yourself. You deserve it.

Don't be afraid to try new things. Eating healthy will give you energy and keep you well for the rest of your life.

Ultimately you should do whatever helps you feel the best, and stick to it. Don't let yourself slide into a degenerative pattern but don't be too hard on yourself. Find a good balance that you're happy with and understand that you want to feel well. You can feel good and be happy about your lifestyle. Choose healthy and live well.

10 BELIEVING IN YOURSELF

There is nothing to lose by trying this out but it is no simple fix. **This takes time**. Do not be so eager as to believe that there really is a miracle pill. There is no such thing as a simple fix. Giving a halfhearted effort will not get you where you need to be in terms of healthiness.

This takes dedication and time, but believe me when I tell you that having your life back is more than worth your time and dedication. Remember, you deserve to be healthy.

As we end, I wanted to address one of the *most* overlooked aspects of healing your body. No matter what it is, you need to believe in yourself. Believe you can be healed. You need to believe you can get better or at least stay positive during the healing process. Start slow, take your time and keep your head up.

Those who do have the right mindset for healing are at great advantage to those who do not. Believing you can be healed speeds up your healing process. It's a very real concept.

On the chemical side of things, your body releases more "happy hormones" when you stay on the positive side. These are beneficial to your body and aid in healing. Additionally, being positive helps you stay motivated and will make you less likely to give up. It will also motivate you to work harder to get better and to share your knowledge with others.

When it comes down to it, staying positive and believing in yourself is one of the most important factors in healing leaky gut because without it, you may not have the will power to get through. Have hope. You will get better!

CONCLUSION

Congratulations! You have gotten to the end of this book. You have learned a lot and taken the first step towards healing your body of Leaky Gut. I commend you for getting this far and encourage you to keep going. There is no limit to what you can do.

The fact that there is truly a way to heal all of these problems is little known and shrouded in speculation. Help me rid the world of Leaky Gut by telling your friends and family. This information is too valuable to keep to yourself. Please share, and help someone in need.

If you would like to stay in touch, feel free to join my email list where I will keep you updated and **send you my *Healthy Living Cookbook* for free**.

You can sign up at: nutritionandhealthyliving.org

Thank you, again, for reading! And congrats again on taking the next best step in your life.

Happy healing and living,
Sage

EXTRAS

Healing Timeline

MONTH 1: Initial Purge: Food and Lifestyle: This is the time to get your eating and lifestyle protocol figured out. Get used to rotating your foods, figure out what foods are causing your reactions, and get on a good diet that makes you feel good. Once you have your food figured out, implement exercise, good sleep habits, reducing stress, etc. Sometimes this might take a little longer than a month, but a month should be a good amount of time to do this. This will also provide enough time eating on the outlined diet to purge toxins from your system, and enough time for you to research and order your supplements. By the end of this you should start feeling your pain go away, have more energy, and start feeling yourself again.

MONTH 2: Final Purge: Supplements: Now is the time to begin taking your supplements. Be sure to watch your reactions and how you feel. If it's too much stress on your body, try waiting a few more weeks before starting the supplements again or lowering the amount you're taking. This is aiding in the continual purge of toxins. It's normal to be extra fatigued when first starting the supplements, but by the end of this month, your body should have purged most toxins from your system and you should be feeling better than you were before.

MONTH 3: Rebirth: L-Glutamine. Now is the time to begin rebuilding your body. Remember, L-Glutamine is a building block in restoring your body back to its normal functioning self but shouldn't be used until your body has purged itself of toxins and is ready to be rebuilt. Again, see how your body reacts to adding in this supplement. If you need to wait a while longer, do. Your body will tell you; it's your best judge. By the end of this you should start feeling back to the way you were before Leaky Gut, or more likely, even better.

MONTH 4: Finality. By this point you should feel great. If you're like me, you might just have a sense of when you know you're healed. If not, you should wait until the end of this month then start introducing some foods back into your diet that you've been avoiding. Watch how you feel, watch your energy levels. If anything feels off stay on the outlined diet until you start feeling you again. By the end of this month, you should be healed. If not, don't be discouraged. We are all different. Our bodies are all different, and yours might just need some extra love. You will get there though!

Step-by-Step Checklist

This checklist is meant to help you follow the outlined information at a pace that fits your lifestyle. The steps are listed in order of what you should do. As you complete a step, move on, but go ahead and take it at your own pace.

Read Chapter 1
Make a list of your symptoms
Read Chapter 3
Create a shopping list and a meal plan
Go shopping for the foods you need
Buy a water-bottle if you don't have one
Begin eating on the outlined diet
Increase water intake
Read Chapter 4
Begin a Food Journal
Read Chapter 2
Remove intolerances from your diet (if you're allergic to too many things to remove, remove the intolerances that cause the biggest reactions)
Begin rotating your foods
Read Chapter 5
Implement exercise
Begin meditating
Evaluate your sleep habits
Reduce Stress
Read Chapter 6
Read Chapter 7
Research Supplements
Order the supplements you will need
Read Chapter 8
Read Chapter 10
Begin taking your supplements
One month later, begin taking L-Glutamine
Read Chapter 9
Compare symptom chart to how you feel now
Congratulations, you should be feeling better!

ABOUT THE AUTHOR

Sage Howard is a wife and mama. She enjoys spending her time with her family, exploring the world, camping, dancing, taking photos and reading good books.

She healed from Leaky Gut four years ago and has since spent much of her time helping those in need also recover from this ailment. Her hope is to show the world that there are alternative and natural ways to treat ailments that are effective and more beneficial to the body and quality of life in the long run than the traditional methods of treatment.

FOUND THIS BOOK HELPFUL?

If you found the information in these pages to be helpful, consider leaving a constructive review. It'll help others on their search for healing.

I read as many reviews as I can, and it usually helps me improve my writing and the information I provide you, so if you feel so inclined go ahead and leave a rating!

Thank you for your support!

Sage

Made in the USA
Middletown, DE
05 December 2017